This book belongs to:

Dedication

This book belongs to anyone who wants to keep track of their medications for health reasons. For anyone who's had difficulty remembering to take their medications, this is for you!

Using This Medication Book

Simply follow the steps listed in the spaces to fill out what medications you're taking, the dosage, what time you took them, side effects, and your physical condition.

📅 DATE		#️⃣ WEEK

💊 NAME	💊 DOSAGE	🕐 TIME	
		:	AM / PM
		:	AM / PM
		:	AM / PM
		:	AM / PM
		:	AM / PM
		:	AM / PM
		:	AM / PM
		:	AM / PM
		:	AM / PM
		:	AM / PM
		:	AM / PM
		:	AM / PM
		:	AM / PM
		:	AM / PM
		:	AM / PM

😷 SIDE EFFECTS	📝 ADDITIONAL NOTES
•	
•	
•	
•	
•	

PHYSICAL CONDITION		
🌙 SLEEP		🥛 WATER
☀️ ENERGY		🏃 ACTIVITY

📅 DATE		# WEEK

💊 NAME	💊 DOSAGE	🕐 TIME
		: AM / PM
		: AM / PM
		: AM / PM
		: AM / PM
		: AM / PM
		: AM / PM
		: AM / PM
		: AM / PM
		: AM / PM
		: AM / PM
		: AM / PM
		: AM / PM
		: AM / PM
		: AM / PM
		: AM / PM

🧑 SIDE EFFECTS	📝 ADDITIONAL NOTES
•	
•	
•	
•	
•	

PHYSICAL CONDITION	
🌙 SLEEP	🥛 WATER
⚡ ENERGY	🏃 ACTIVITY

📅 DATE		# WEEK

💊 NAME	💊 DOSAGE	🕐 TIME
		: AM / PM
		: AM / PM
		: AM / PM
		: AM / PM
		: AM / PM
		: AM / PM
		: AM / PM
		: AM / PM
		: AM / PM
		: AM / PM
		: AM / PM
		: AM / PM
		: AM / PM
		: AM / PM
		: AM / PM

🧠 SIDE EFFECTS	📝 ADDITIONAL NOTES
.	
.	
.	
.	
.	

PHYSICAL CONDITION	
🌙 SLEEP	💧 WATER
⚡ ENERGY	🏃 ACTIVITY

📅 DATE		# WEEK	

💊 NAME	💊 DOSAGE	🕐 TIME	
		:	AM / PM
		:	AM / PM
		:	AM / PM
		:	AM / PM
		:	AM / PM
		:	AM / PM
		:	AM / PM
		:	AM / PM
		:	AM / PM
		:	AM / PM
		:	AM / PM
		:	AM / PM
		:	AM / PM
		:	AM / PM
		:	AM / PM

🧠 SIDE EFFECTS	📝 ADDITIONAL NOTES
•	
•	
•	
•	
•	

PHYSICAL CONDITION	
🌙 SLEEP	🥛 WATER
⚡ ENERGY	🏃 ACTIVITY

📅 DATE		# WEEK	

💊 NAME	🪴 DOSAGE	🕐 TIME	
		:	AM / PM
		:	AM / PM
		:	AM / PM
		:	AM / PM
		:	AM / PM
		:	AM / PM
		:	AM / PM
		:	AM / PM
		:	AM / PM
		:	AM / PM
		:	AM / PM
		:	AM / PM
		:	AM / PM
		:	AM / PM
		:	AM / PM

🤕 SIDE EFFECTS	📝 ADDITIONAL NOTES
•	
•	
•	
•	
•	

PHYSICAL CONDITION			
🌙 SLEEP	⬜⬜⬜⬜⬜	🥤 WATER	⬜⬜⬜⬜⬜
☀️ ENERGY	⬜⬜⬜⬜⬜	🏃 ACTIVITY	⬜⬜⬜⬜⬜

📅 DATE		# WEEK

💊 NAME	💊 DOSAGE	🕐 TIME
		: AM / PM
		: AM / PM
		: AM / PM
		: AM / PM
		: AM / PM
		: AM / PM
		: AM / PM
		: AM / PM
		: AM / PM
		: AM / PM
		: AM / PM
		: AM / PM
		: AM / PM
		: AM / PM
		: AM / PM

🧠 SIDE EFFECTS	📝 ADDITIONAL NOTES
•	
•	
•	
•	
•	

PHYSICAL CONDITION	
🌙 SLEEP	🥤 WATER
☀️ ENERGY	🏃 ACTIVITY

📅 DATE		# WEEK	

💊 NAME	🌱 DOSAGE	🕐 TIME	
		:	AM / PM
		:	AM / PM
		:	AM / PM
		:	AM / PM
		:	AM / PM
		:	AM / PM
		:	AM / PM
		:	AM / PM
		:	AM / PM
		:	AM / PM
		:	AM / PM
		:	AM / PM
		:	AM / PM
		:	AM / PM
		:	AM / PM

🤕 SIDE EFFECTS	📝 ADDITIONAL NOTES
•	
•	
•	
•	
•	

PHYSICAL CONDITION	
🌙 SLEEP	🥛 WATER
☀ ENERGY	🏃 ACTIVITY

DATE	WEEK

🔖 NAME	💧 DOSAGE	🕐 TIME
		: AM / PM
		: AM / PM
		: AM / PM
		: AM / PM
		: AM / PM
		: AM / PM
		: AM / PM
		: AM / PM
		: AM / PM
		: AM / PM
		: AM / PM
		: AM / PM
		: AM / PM
		: AM / PM
		: AM / PM

🤕 SIDE EFFECTS	📝 ADDITIONAL NOTES
•	
•	
•	
•	
•	

PHYSICAL CONDITION	
🌙 SLEEP	🥛 WATER
⚡ ENERGY	🏃 ACTIVITY

📅 DATE		# WEEK	

💊 NAME	🌱 DOSAGE	🕐 TIME	
		:	AM / PM
		:	AM / PM
		:	AM / PM
		:	AM / PM
		:	AM / PM
		:	AM / PM
		:	AM / PM
		:	AM / PM
		:	AM / PM
		:	AM / PM
		:	AM / PM
		:	AM / PM
		:	AM / PM
		:	AM / PM
		:	AM / PM

🗣 SIDE EFFECTS	📝 ADDITIONAL NOTES
•	
•	
•	
•	
•	

PHYSICAL CONDITION	
🌙 SLEEP	💧 WATER
⚡ ENERGY	🏃 ACTIVITY

📅 DATE		# WEEK

💊 NAME	💊 DOSAGE	⏰ TIME
		: AM / PM
		: AM / PM
		: AM / PM
		: AM / PM
		: AM / PM
		: AM / PM
		: AM / PM
		: AM / PM
		: AM / PM
		: AM / PM
		: AM / PM
		: AM / PM
		: AM / PM
		: AM / PM
		: AM / PM

🧠 SIDE EFFECTS	📝 ADDITIONAL NOTES
•	
•	
•	
•	
•	

PHYSICAL CONDITION	
🌙 SLEEP ▭▭▭▭▭	🥛 WATER ▭▭▭▭▭
⚡ ENERGY ▭▭▭▭▭	🏃 ACTIVITY ▭▭▭▭▭

📅 DATE		# WEEK

💊 NAME	💊 DOSAGE	⏱ TIME
		: AM / PM
		: AM / PM
		: AM / PM
		: AM / PM
		: AM / PM
		: AM / PM
		: AM / PM
		: AM / PM
		: AM / PM
		: AM / PM
		: AM / PM
		: AM / PM
		: AM / PM
		: AM / PM
		: AM / PM

🧠 SIDE EFFECTS	📝 ADDITIONAL NOTES
•	
•	
•	
•	
•	

PHYSICAL CONDITION			
🌙 SLEEP	⬜⬜⬜⬜⬜	💧 WATER	⬜⬜⬜⬜⬜
⚡ ENERGY	⬜⬜⬜⬜⬜	🏃 ACTIVITY	⬜⬜⬜⬜⬜

📅 DATE		# WEEK

💊 NAME	💧 DOSAGE	🕐 TIME
		: AM / PM
		: AM / PM
		: AM / PM
		: AM / PM
		: AM / PM
		: AM / PM
		: AM / PM
		: AM / PM
		: AM / PM
		: AM / PM
		: AM / PM
		: AM / PM
		: AM / PM
		: AM / PM
		: AM / PM

🧠 SIDE EFFECTS	📝 ADDITIONAL NOTES
•	
•	
•	
•	
•	

PHYSICAL CONDITION	
🌙 SLEEP	🥤 WATER
☀️ ENERGY	🏃 ACTIVITY

📅 DATE		# WEEK

💊 NAME	🪴 DOSAGE	🕐 TIME
		: AM / PM
		: AM / PM
		: AM / PM
		: AM / PM
		: AM / PM
		: AM / PM
		: AM / PM
		: AM / PM
		: AM / PM
		: AM / PM
		: AM / PM
		: AM / PM
		: AM / PM
		: AM / PM
		: AM / PM
		: AM / PM

🤕 SIDE EFFECTS	📝 ADDITIONAL NOTES
•	
•	
•	
•	
•	

PHYSICAL CONDITION			
🌙 SLEEP	▭▭▭▭▭	🥛 WATER	▭▭▭▭▭
☀️ ENERGY	▭▭▭▭▭	🏃 ACTIVITY	▭▭▭▭▭

▦ DATE		# WEEK

⬭ NAME	⬭ DOSAGE	⬭ TIME
		: AM / PM
		: AM / PM
		: AM / PM
		: AM / PM
		: AM / PM
		: AM / PM
		: AM / PM
		: AM / PM
		: AM / PM
		: AM / PM
		: AM / PM
		: AM / PM
		: AM / PM
		: AM / PM
		: AM / PM

⬭ SIDE EFFECTS	⬭ ADDITIONAL NOTES
•	
•	
•	
•	
•	

PHYSICAL CONDITION	
☾ SLEEP ▭▭▭▭▭	⬭ WATER ▭▭▭▭▭
☀ ENERGY ▭▭▭▭▭	⬭ ACTIVITY ▭▭▭▭▭

📅 DATE		# WEEK

💊 NAME	🌱 DOSAGE	🕐 TIME	
		:	AM / PM
		:	AM / PM
		:	AM / PM
		:	AM / PM
		:	AM / PM
		:	AM / PM
		:	AM / PM
		:	AM / PM
		:	AM / PM
		:	AM / PM
		:	AM / PM
		:	AM / PM
		:	AM / PM
		:	AM / PM
		:	AM / PM

🗣 SIDE EFFECTS	📝 ADDITIONAL NOTES
•	
•	
•	
•	
•	

PHYSICAL CONDITION	
🌙 SLEEP	🥛 WATER
⚡ ENERGY	🏃 ACTIVITY

📅 DATE		#️⃣ WEEK

💊 NAME	🌱 DOSAGE	🕐 TIME	
		:	AM / PM
		:	AM / PM
		:	AM / PM
		:	AM / PM
		:	AM / PM
		:	AM / PM
		:	AM / PM
		:	AM / PM
		:	AM / PM
		:	AM / PM
		:	AM / PM
		:	AM / PM
		:	AM / PM
		:	AM / PM
		:	AM / PM

🧠 SIDE EFFECTS	📝 ADDITIONAL NOTES
•	
•	
•	
•	
•	

PHYSICAL CONDITION			
🌙 SLEEP	▭▭▭▭▭	🥛 WATER	▭▭▭▭▭
⚡ ENERGY	▭▭▭▭▭	🏃 ACTIVITY	▭▭▭▭▭

📅 DATE		#️⃣ WEEK

💊 NAME	🌱 DOSAGE	⏰ TIME
		: AM / PM
		: AM / PM
		: AM / PM
		: AM / PM
		: AM / PM
		: AM / PM
		: AM / PM
		: AM / PM
		: AM / PM
		: AM / PM
		: AM / PM
		: AM / PM
		: AM / PM
		: AM / PM
		: AM / PM

🧠 SIDE EFFECTS	📝 ADDITIONAL NOTES
•	
•	
•	
•	
•	

PHYSICAL CONDITION	
🌙 SLEEP ⬜⬜⬜⬜⬜	🥛 WATER ⬜⬜⬜⬜⬜
⚡ ENERGY ⬜⬜⬜⬜⬜	🏃 ACTIVITY ⬜⬜⬜⬜⬜

📅 DATE		# WEEK	

💊 NAME	💊 DOSAGE	🕐 TIME	
		:	AM / PM
		:	AM / PM
		:	AM / PM
		:	AM / PM
		:	AM / PM
		:	AM / PM
		:	AM / PM
		:	AM / PM
		:	AM / PM
		:	AM / PM
		:	AM / PM
		:	AM / PM
		:	∧M / PM
		:	AM / PM
		:	AM / PM

🧠 SIDE EFFECTS	📝 ADDITIONAL NOTES
•	
•	
•	
•	
•	

PHYSICAL CONDITION			
🌙 SLEEP	▭▭▭▭▭	🥤 WATER	▭▭▭▭▭
⚡ ENERGY	▭▭▭▭▭	🏃 ACTIVITY	▭▭▭▭▭

📅 DATE		#️⃣ WEEK

💊 NAME	💊 DOSAGE	💊 TIME	
		:	AM / PM
		:	AM / PM
		:	AM / PM
		:	AM / PM
		:	AM / PM
		:	AM / PM
		:	AM / PM
		:	AM / PM
		:	AM / PM
		:	AM / PM
		:	AM / PM
		:	AM / PM
		:	AM / PM
		:	AM / PM
		:	AM / PM

🤕 SIDE EFFECTS	📝 ADDITIONAL NOTES
•	
•	
•	
•	
•	

PHYSICAL CONDITION		
🌙 SLEEP	⬜⬜⬜⬜⬜	🥛 WATER	⬜⬜⬜⬜⬜
⚡ ENERGY	⬜⬜⬜⬜⬜	🏃 ACTIVITY	⬜⬜⬜⬜⬜

📅 DATE	# WEEK

💊 NAME	💊 DOSAGE	🕐 TIME
		: AM / PM
		: AM / PM
		: AM / PM
		: AM / PM
		: AM / PM
		: AM / PM
		: AM / PM
		: AM / PM
		: AM / PM
		: AM / PM
		: AM / PM
		: AM / PM
		: AM / PM
		: AM / PM
		: AM / PM

🧠 SIDE EFFECTS	📝 ADDITIONAL NOTES
•	
•	
•	
•	
•	

PHYSICAL CONDITION

🌙 SLEEP	⬭⬭⬭⬭	🥛 WATER	⬭⬭⬭⬭
☀️ ENERGY	⬭⬭⬭⬭	🏃 ACTIVITY	⬭⬭⬭⬭

📅 DATE		# WEEK

💊 NAME	💊 DOSAGE	🕑 TIME
		: AM / PM
		: AM / PM
		: AM / PM
		: AM / PM
		: AM / PM
		: AM / PM
		: AM / PM
		: AM / PM
		: AM / PM
		: AM / PM
		: AM / PM
		: AM / PM
		: AM / PM
		: AM / PM
		: AM / PM

🧠 SIDE EFFECTS	📝 ADDITIONAL NOTES
•	
•	
•	
•	
•	

PHYSICAL CONDITION	
🌙 SLEEP	💧 WATER
⚡ ENERGY	🏃 ACTIVITY

📅 DATE		# WEEK

💊 NAME	🌱 DOSAGE	🕐 TIME
		: AM / PM
		: AM / PM
		: AM / PM
		: AM / PM
		: AM / PM
		: AM / PM
		: AM / PM
		: AM / PM
		: AM / PM
		: AM / PM
		: AM / PM
		: AM / PM
		: AM / PM
		: AM / PM
		: AM / PM

🧠 SIDE EFFECTS	📝 ADDITIONAL NOTES
•	
•	
•	
•	
•	

PHYSICAL CONDITION	
🌙 SLEEP ▭▭▭▭▭	🥛 WATER ▭▭▭▭▭
☀️ ENERGY ▭▭▭▭▭	🏃 ACTIVITY ▭▭▭▭▭

📅 DATE		# WEEK	

💊 NAME	🌱 DOSAGE	🕐 TIME	
		:	AM / PM
		:	AM / PM
		:	AM / PM
		:	AM / PM
		:	AM / PM
		:	AM / PM
		:	AM / PM
		:	AM / PM
		:	AM / PM
		:	AM / PM
		:	AM / PM
		:	AM / PM
		:	AM / PM
		:	AM / PM
		:	AM / PM

🤕 SIDE EFFECTS	📝 ADDITIONAL NOTES
•	
•	
•	
•	
•	

PHYSICAL CONDITION			
🌙 SLEEP	⬜⬜⬜⬜⬜	🥛 WATER	⬜⬜⬜⬜⬜
⚡ ENERGY	⬜⬜⬜⬜⬜	🏃 ACTIVITY	⬜⬜⬜⬜⬜

📅 DATE		# WEEK

💊 NAME	💊 DOSAGE	⏰ TIME	
		:	AM / PM
		:	AM / PM
		:	AM / PM
		:	AM / PM
		:	AM / PM
		:	AM / PM
		:	AM / PM
		:	AM / PM
		:	AM / PM
		:	AM / PM
		:	AM / PM
		:	AM / PM
		:	AM / PM
		:	AM / PM
		:	AM / PM

🤕 SIDE EFFECTS	📝 ADDITIONAL NOTES
•	
•	
•	
•	
•	

PHYSICAL CONDITION			
🌙 SLEEP	☐☐☐☐☐	🥛 WATER	☐☐☐☐☐
⚡ ENERGY	☐☐☐☐☐	🏃 ACTIVITY	☐☐☐☐☐

📅 DATE		# WEEK

💊 NAME	💊 DOSAGE	🕐 TIME
		: AM / PM
		: AM / PM
		: AM / PM
		: AM / PM
		: AM / PM
		: AM / PM
		: AM / PM
		: AM / PM
		: AM / PM
		: AM / PM
		: AM / PM
		: AM / PM
		: AM / PM
		: AM / PM
		: AM / PM

🗣 SIDE EFFECTS	📝 ADDITIONAL NOTES
•	
•	
•	
•	
•	

PHYSICAL CONDITION

🌙 SLEEP	☐☐☐☐☐	🥛 WATER	☐☐☐☐☐
⚡ ENERGY	☐☐☐☐☐	🏃 ACTIVITY	☐☐☐☐☐

📅 DATE		# WEEK

💊 NAME	💊 DOSAGE	💊 TIME
		: AM / PM
		: AM / PM
		: AM / PM
		: AM / PM
		: AM / PM
		: AM / PM
		: AM / PM
		: AM / PM
		: AM / PM
		: AM / PM
		: AM / PM
		: AM / PM
		: AM / PM
		: AM / PM
		: AM / PM

🤕 SIDE EFFECTS	📝 ADDITIONAL NOTES
•	
•	
•	
•	
•	

PHYSICAL CONDITION			
🌙 SLEEP	☐☐☐☐☐	🥛 WATER	☐☐☐☐☐
⚡ ENERGY	☐☐☐☐☐	🏃 ACTIVITY	☐☐☐☐☐

📅 DATE		# WEEK	

💊 NAME	💊 DOSAGE	🕐 TIME	
		:	AM / PM
		:	AM / PM
		:	AM / PM
		:	AM / PM
		:	AM / PM
		:	AM / PM
		:	AM / PM
		:	AM / PM
		:	AM / PM
		:	AM / PM
		:	AM / PM
		:	AM / PM
		:	AM / PM
		:	AM / PM
		:	AM / PM

🗯 SIDE EFFECTS	📝 ADDITIONAL NOTES
•	
•	
•	
•	
•	

PHYSICAL CONDITION			
🌙 SLEEP	⬜⬜⬜⬜⬜	🥤 WATER	⬜⬜⬜⬜⬜
⚡ ENERGY	⬜⬜⬜⬜⬜	🏃 ACTIVITY	⬜⬜⬜⬜⬜

📅 DATE	# WEEK

💊 NAME	🌿 DOSAGE	🕐 TIME
		: AM / PM
		: AM / PM
		: AM / PM
		: AM / PM
		: AM / PM
		: AM / PM
		: AM / PM
		: AM / PM
		: AM / PM
		: AM / PM
		: AM / PM
		: AM / PM
		: AM / PM
		: AM / PM
		: AM / PM

🙂 SIDE EFFECTS	📝 ADDITIONAL NOTES
•	
•	
•	
•	
•	

PHYSICAL CONDITION	
🌙 SLEEP	🥛 WATER
⚡ ENERGY	🏃 ACTIVITY

📅 DATE		# WEEK	

💊 NAME	💊 DOSAGE	🕐 TIME	
		:	AM / PM
		:	AM / PM
		:	AM / PM
		:	AM / PM
		:	AM / PM
		:	AM / PM
		:	AM / PM
		:	AM / PM
		:	AM / PM
		:	AM / PM
		:	AM / PM
		:	AM / PM
		:	AM / PM
		:	AM / PM
		:	AM / PM

🧠 SIDE EFFECTS	📝 ADDITIONAL NOTES
•	
•	
•	
•	
•	

PHYSICAL CONDITION			
🌙 SLEEP	⬜⬜⬜⬜⬜	🥛 WATER	⬜⬜⬜⬜⬜
⚡ ENERGY	⬜⬜⬜⬜⬜	🏃 ACTIVITY	⬜⬜⬜⬜⬜

📅 DATE		# WEEK

💊 NAME	🧪 DOSAGE	🕑 TIME
		: AM / PM
		: AM / PM
		: AM / PM
		: AM / PM
		: AM / PM
		: AM / PM
		: AM / PM
		: AM / PM
		: AM / PM
		: AM / PM
		: AM / PM
		: AM / PM
		: AM / PM
		: AM / PM
		: AM / PM

🧠 SIDE EFFECTS	📝 ADDITIONAL NOTES
•	
•	
•	
•	
•	

PHYSICAL CONDITION	
🌙 SLEEP	🥛 WATER
⚡ ENERGY	🏃 ACTIVITY

📅 DATE	# WEEK

💊 NAME	🌱 DOSAGE	🕐 TIME	
		:	AM / PM
		:	AM / PM
		:	AM / PM
		:	AM / PM
		:	AM / PM
		:	AM / PM
		:	AM / PM
		:	AM / PM
		:	AM / PM
		:	AM / PM
		:	AM / PM
		:	AM / PM
		:	AM / PM
		:	AM / PM
		:	AM / PM

🧠 SIDE EFFECTS	📝 ADDITIONAL NOTES
•	
•	
•	
•	
•	

PHYSICAL CONDITION	
☾ SLEEP	🥛 WATER
⚡ ENERGY	🏃 ACTIVITY

📅 DATE		# WEEK

💊 NAME	🌱 DOSAGE	🕐 TIME
		: AM / PM
		: AM / PM
		: AM / PM
		: AM / PM
		: AM / PM
		: AM / PM
		: AM / PM
		: AM / PM
		: AM / PM
		: AM / PM
		: AM / PM
		: AM / PM
		: AM / PM
		: AM / PM
		: AM / PM

🤕 SIDE EFFECTS	📝 ADDITIONAL NOTES
•	
•	
•	
•	
•	

PHYSICAL CONDITION			
🌙 SLEEP	▭▭▭▭▭	🥛 WATER	▭▭▭▭▭
☀️ ENERGY	▭▭▭▭▭	🏃 ACTIVITY	▭▭▭▭▭

📅 DATE		#️⃣ WEEK

💊 NAME	💊 DOSAGE	🕑 TIME
		: AM / PM
		: AM / PM
		: AM / PM
		: AM / PM
		: AM / PM
		: AM / PM
		: AM / PM
		: AM / PM
		: AM / PM
		: AM / PM
		: AM / PM
		: AM / PM
		: AM / PM
		: AM / PM
		: AM / PM

🧠 SIDE EFFECTS	📝 ADDITIONAL NOTES
•	
•	
•	
•	
•	

PHYSICAL CONDITION			
🌙 SLEEP	☐☐☐☐☐	🥛 WATER	☐☐☐☐☐
⚡ ENERGY	☐☐☐☐☐	🏃 ACTIVITY	☐☐☐☐☐

📅 DATE		#️⃣ WEEK	

💊 NAME	🌱 DOSAGE	🕐 TIME	
		:	AM / PM
		:	AM / PM
		:	AM / PM
		:	AM / PM
		:	AM / PM
		:	AM / PM
		:	AM / PM
		:	AM / PM
		:	AM / PM
		:	AM / PM
		:	AM / PM
		:	AM / PM
		:	AM / PM
		:	AM / PM
		:	AM / PM

🗣 SIDE EFFECTS	📝 ADDITIONAL NOTES
•	
•	
•	
•	
•	

PHYSICAL CONDITION			
🌙 SLEEP	▭▭▭▭▭	🥛 WATER	▭▭▭▭▭
☀ ENERGY	▭▭▭▭▭	🏃 ACTIVITY	▭▭▭▭▭

📅 DATE		# WEEK

💊 NAME	🧴 DOSAGE	🕐 TIME	
		:	AM / PM
		:	AM / PM
		:	AM / PM
		:	AM / PM
		:	AM / PM
		:	AM / PM
		:	AM / PM
		:	AM / PM
		:	AM / PM
		:	AM / PM
		:	AM / PM
		:	AM / PM
		:	AM / PM
		:	AM / PM
		:	AM / PM

🧠 SIDE EFFECTS	📝 ADDITIONAL NOTES
•	
•	
•	
•	
•	

PHYSICAL CONDITION	
🌙 SLEEP	💧 WATER
⚡ ENERGY	🏃 ACTIVITY

📅 DATE		# WEEK

💊 NAME	💊 DOSAGE	🕐 TIME
		: AM / PM
		: AM / PM
		: AM / PM
		: AM / PM
		: AM / PM
		: AM / PM
		: AM / PM
		: AM / PM
		: AM / PM
		: AM / PM
		: AM / PM
		: AM / PM
		: AM / PM
		: AM / PM
		: AM / PM

🧠 SIDE EFFECTS	📝 ADDITIONAL NOTES
•	
•	
•	
•	
•	

PHYSICAL CONDITION	
🌙 SLEEP	🥤 WATER
☀️ ENERGY	🏃 ACTIVITY

📅 DATE		# WEEK

💊 NAME	🧪 DOSAGE	🕐 TIME	
		:	AM / PM
		:	AM / PM
		:	AM / PM
		:	AM / PM
		:	AM / PM
		:	AM / PM
		:	AM / PM
		:	AM / PM
		:	AM / PM
		:	AM / PM
		:	AM / PM
		:	AM / PM
		:	AM / PM
		:	AM / PM
		:	AM / PM

🧠 SIDE EFFECTS	📝 ADDITIONAL NOTES
·	
·	
·	
·	
·	

PHYSICAL CONDITION	
🌙 SLEEP	🥤 WATER
⚡ ENERGY	🏃 ACTIVITY

📅 DATE		# WEEK

💊 NAME	💊 DOSAGE	⏰ TIME
		: AM / PM
		: AM / PM
		: AM / PM
		: AM / PM
		: AM / PM
		: AM / PM
		: AM / PM
		: AM / PM
		: AM / PM
		: AM / PM
		: AM / PM
		: AM / PM
		: AM / PM
		: AM / PM
		: AM / PM

🧠 SIDE EFFECTS	📝 ADDITIONAL NOTES
•	
•	
•	
•	
•	

PHYSICAL CONDITION			
🌙 SLEEP	⬭⬜⬜⬜⬜	🥛 WATER	⬭⬜⬜⬜⬜
⚡ ENERGY	⬭⬜⬜⬜⬜	🏃 ACTIVITY	⬭⬜⬜⬜⬜

📅 DATE		# WEEK

💊 NAME	💊 DOSAGE	🕐 TIME
		: AM / PM
		: AM / PM
		: AM / PM
		: AM / PM
		: AM / PM
		: AM / PM
		: AM / PM
		: AM / PM
		: AM / PM
		: AM / PM
		: AM / PM
		: AM / PM
		: AM / PM
		: AM / PM
		: AM / PM

🧠 SIDE EFFECTS	📝 ADDITIONAL NOTES
•	
•	
•	
•	
•	

PHYSICAL CONDITION		
🌙 SLEEP		🥛 WATER
⚡ ENERGY		🏃 ACTIVITY

📅 DATE		# WEEK

💊 NAME	💊 DOSAGE	🕐 TIME
		: AM / PM
		: AM / PM
		: AM / PM
		: AM / PM
		: AM / PM
		: AM / PM
		: AM / PM
		: AM / PM
		: AM / PM
		: AM / PM
		: AM / PM
		: AM / PM
		: AM / PM
		: AM / PM
		: AM / PM

🧠 SIDE EFFECTS	📝 ADDITIONAL NOTES
·	
·	
·	
·	
·	

PHYSICAL CONDITION	
🌙 SLEEP	🥛 WATER
⚡ ENERGY	🏃 ACTIVITY

📅 DATE		# WEEK

💊 NAME	🌱 DOSAGE	💊 TIME
		: AM / PM
		: AM / PM
		: AM / PM
		: AM / PM
		: AM / PM
		: AM / PM
		: AM / PM
		: AM / PM
		: AM / PM
		: AM / PM
		: AM / PM
		: AM / PM
		: AM / PM
		: AM / PM
		: AM / PM

🧠 SIDE EFFECTS	📝 ADDITIONAL NOTES
•	
•	
•	
•	
•	

PHYSICAL CONDITION	
🌙 SLEEP	🥛 WATER
⚡ ENERGY	🏃 ACTIVITY

📅 DATE	# WEEK

💊 NAME	💊 DOSAGE	🕐 TIME
		: AM / PM
		: AM / PM
		: AM / PM
		: AM / PM
		: AM / PM
		: AM / PM
		: AM / PM
		: AM / PM
		: AM / PM
		: AM / PM
		: AM / PM
		: AM / PM
		: AM / PM
		: AM / PM
		: AM / PM

🧑 SIDE EFFECTS	📝 ADDITIONAL NOTES
•	
•	
•	
•	
•	

PHYSICAL CONDITION

🌙 SLEEP	⬡⬡⬡⬡	🥛 WATER	⬡⬡⬡⬡
☀️ ENERGY	⬡⬡⬡⬡	🏃 ACTIVITY	⬡⬡⬡⬡

📅 DATE		# WEEK

💊 NAME	💊 DOSAGE	🕐 TIME
		: AM / PM
		: AM / PM
		: AM / PM
		: AM / PM
		: AM / PM
		: AM / PM
		: AM / PM
		: AM / PM
		: AM / PM
		: AM / PM
		: AM / PM
		: AM / PM
		: AM / PM
		: AM / PM
		: AM / PM

🧠 SIDE EFFECTS	📝 ADDITIONAL NOTES
•	
•	
•	
•	
•	

PHYSICAL CONDITION		
🌙 SLEEP	☐☐☐☐☐	
☀ ENERGY	☐☐☐☐☐	
🥛 WATER	☐☐☐☐☐	
🏃 ACTIVITY	☐☐☐☐☐	

📅 DATE	# WEEK

💊 NAME	🌱 DOSAGE	⏰ TIME
		: AM / PM
		: AM / PM
		: AM / PM
		: AM / PM
		: AM / PM
		: AM / PM
		: AM / PM
		: AM / PM
		: AM / PM
		: AM / PM
		: AM / PM
		: AM / PM
		: AM / PM
		: AM / PM
		: AM / PM

🤕 SIDE EFFECTS	📝 ADDITIONAL NOTES
•	
•	
•	
•	
•	

PHYSICAL CONDITION	
🌙 SLEEP	🥛 WATER
☀ ENERGY	🏃 ACTIVITY

📅 DATE		# WEEK

💊 NAME	💊 DOSAGE	🕐 TIME
		: AM / PM
		: AM / PM
		: AM / PM
		: AM / PM
		: AM / PM
		: AM / PM
		: AM / PM
		: AM / PM
		: AM / PM
		: AM / PM
		: AM / PM
		: AM / PM
		: AM / PM
		: AM / PM
		: AM / PM

🗣 SIDE EFFECTS	📝 ADDITIONAL NOTES
•	
•	
•	
•	
•	

PHYSICAL CONDITION	
🌙 SLEEP	🥛 WATER
🔅 ENERGY	🏃 ACTIVITY

📅 DATE		# WEEK

💊 NAME	💊 DOSAGE	🕐 TIME
		: AM / PM
		: AM / PM
		: AM / PM
		: AM / PM
		: AM / PM
		: AM / PM
		: AM / PM
		: AM / PM
		: AM / PM
		: AM / PM
		: AM / PM
		: AM / PM
		: AM / PM
		: AM / PM
		: AM / PM

🧠 SIDE EFFECTS	📝 ADDITIONAL NOTES
•	
•	
•	
•	
•	

PHYSICAL CONDITION	
🌙 SLEEP ▭▭▭▭▭	🥛 WATER ▭▭▭▭▭
⚡ ENERGY ▭▭▭▭▭	🏃 ACTIVITY ▭▭▭▭▭

📅 DATE		# WEEK

💊 NAME	🌱 DOSAGE	⏰ TIME
		: AM / PM
		: AM / PM
		: AM / PM
		: AM / PM
		: AM / PM
		: AM / PM
		: AM / PM
		: AM / PM
		: AM / PM
		: AM / PM
		: AM / PM
		: AM / PM
		: AM / PM
		: AM / PM
		: AM / PM

🧠 SIDE EFFECTS	📝 ADDITIONAL NOTES
•	
•	
•	
•	
•	

PHYSICAL CONDITION			
🌙 SLEEP	⬭⬭⬭⬭⬭	🥛 WATER	⬭⬭⬭⬭⬭
⚡ ENERGY	⬭⬭⬭⬭⬭	🏃 ACTIVITY	⬭⬭⬭⬭⬭

📅 DATE		# WEEK

💊 NAME	🧪 DOSAGE	🕐 TIME
		: AM / PM
		: AM / PM
		: AM / PM
		: AM / PM
		: AM / PM
		: AM / PM
		: AM / PM
		: AM / PM
		: AM / PM
		: AM / PM
		: AM / PM
		: AM / PM
		: AM / PM
		: AM / PM
		: AM / PM

🤕 SIDE EFFECTS	📝 ADDITIONAL NOTES
•	
•	
•	
•	
•	

PHYSICAL CONDITION		
🌙 SLEEP		🥛 WATER
⚡ ENERGY		🏃 ACTIVITY

📅 DATE		# WEEK

💊 NAME	💊 DOSAGE	🕐 TIME
		: AM / PM
		: AM / PM
		: AM / PM
		: AM / PM
		: AM / PM
		: AM / PM
		: AM / PM
		: AM / PM
		: AM / PM
		: AM / PM
		: AM / PM
		: AM / PM
		: AM / PM
		: AM / PM
		: AM / PM

😷 SIDE EFFECTS	📝 ADDITIONAL NOTES
•	
•	
•	
•	
•	

PHYSICAL CONDITION		
🌙 SLEEP	[＿＿＿＿＿]	WATER [＿＿＿＿＿]
⚡ ENERGY	[＿＿＿＿＿]	🏃 ACTIVITY [＿＿＿＿＿]

📅 DATE	# WEEK

💊 NAME	🧴 DOSAGE	🕐 TIME
		: ___ AM / PM
		: ___ AM / PM
		: ___ AM / PM
		: ___ AM / PM
		: ___ AM / PM
		: ___ AM / PM
		: ___ AM / PM
		: ___ AM / PM
		: ___ AM / PM
		: ___ AM / PM
		: ___ AM / PM
		: ___ AM / PM
		: ___ AM / PM
		: ___ AM / PM
		: ___ AM / PM

🪣 SIDE EFFECTS	📝 ADDITIONAL NOTES
•	
•	
•	
•	
•	

PHYSICAL CONDITION	
🌙 SLEEP	🥛 WATER
⚡ ENERGY	🏃 ACTIVITY

📅 DATE	# WEEK

💊 NAME	🧴 DOSAGE	⏰ TIME	
		:	AM / PM
		:	AM / PM
		:	AM / PM
		:	AM / PM
		:	AM / PM
		:	AM / PM
		:	AM / PM
		:	AM / PM
		:	AM / PM
		:	AM / PM
		:	AM / PM
		:	AM / PM
		:	AM / PM
		:	AM / PM
		:	AM / PM

🤕 SIDE EFFECTS	📝 ADDITIONAL NOTES
•	
•	
•	
•	
•	

PHYSICAL CONDITION			
🌙 SLEEP	☐☐☐☐☐	🥛 WATER	☐☐☐☐☐
☀ ENERGY	☐☐☐☐☐	🏃 ACTIVITY	☐☐☐☐☐

📅 DATE		# WEEK

💊 NAME	💊 DOSAGE	🕐 TIME
		: AM / PM
		: AM / PM
		: AM / PM
		: AM / PM
		: AM / PM
		: AM / PM
		: AM / PM
		: AM / PM
		: AM / PM
		: AM / PM
		: AM / PM
		: AM / PM
		: AM / PM
		: AM / PM
		: AM / PM

🧠 SIDE EFFECTS	📝 ADDITIONAL NOTES
•	
•	
•	
•	
•	

PHYSICAL CONDITION	
🌙 SLEEP	🥤 WATER
☀️ ENERGY	🏃 ACTIVITY

📅 DATE		# WEEK

💊 NAME	💊 DOSAGE	🕐 TIME
		: AM / PM
		: AM / PM
		: AM / PM
		: AM / PM
		: AM / PM
		: AM / PM
		: AM / PM
		: AM / PM
		: AM / PM
		: AM / PM
		: AM / PM
		: AM / PM
		: AM / PM
		: AM / PM
		: AM / PM

😷 SIDE EFFECTS	📝 ADDITIONAL NOTES
•	
•	
•	
•	
•	

PHYSICAL CONDITION			
🌙 SLEEP	⬜⬜⬜⬜⬜	🥤 WATER	⬜⬜⬜⬜⬜
⚡ ENERGY	⬜⬜⬜⬜⬜	🏃 ACTIVITY	⬜⬜⬜⬜⬜

📅 DATE		#️⃣ WEEK

💊 NAME	🌱 DOSAGE	🕐 TIME
		: AM / PM
		: AM / PM
		: AM / PM
		: AM / PM
		: AM / PM
		: AM / PM
		: AM / PM
		: AM / PM
		: AM / PM
		: AM / PM
		: AM / PM
		: AM / PM
		: AM / PM
		: AM / PM
		: AM / PM

🗣 SIDE EFFECTS	📝 ADDITIONAL NOTES
•	
•	
•	
•	
•	

PHYSICAL CONDITION	
🌙 SLEEP	🥛 WATER
⚡ ENERGY	🏃 ACTIVITY

📅 DATE		# WEEK	

💊 NAME	🌱 DOSAGE	⏱ TIME	
		:	AM / PM
		:	AM / PM
		:	AM / PM
		:	AM / PM
		:	AM / PM
		:	AM / PM
		:	AM / PM
		:	AM / PM
		:	AM / PM
		:	AM / PM
		:	AM / PM
		:	AM / PM
		:	AM / PM
		:	AM / PM
		:	AM / PM

🧠 SIDE EFFECTS	📝 ADDITIONAL NOTES
•	
•	
•	
•	
•	

PHYSICAL CONDITION			
🌙 SLEEP	⬜⬜⬜⬜⬜	🥛 WATER	⬜⬜⬜⬜⬜
⚡ ENERGY	⬜⬜⬜⬜⬜	🏃 ACTIVITY	⬜⬜⬜⬜⬜

📅 DATE		# WEEK

💊 NAME	🥄 DOSAGE	🕐 TIME
		: AM / PM
		: AM / PM
		: AM / PM
		: AM / PM
		: AM / PM
		: AM / PM
		: AM / PM
		: AM / PM
		: AM / PM
		: AM / PM
		: AM / PM
		: AM / PM
		: AM / PM
		: AM / PM
		: AM / PM

🧠 SIDE EFFECTS	📝 ADDITIONAL NOTES
•	
•	
•	
•	
•	

PHYSICAL CONDITION	
🌙 SLEEP ⬭⬜⬜⬜⬭	🥤 WATER ⬭⬜⬜⬜⬭
⚡ ENERGY ⬭⬜⬜⬜⬭	🏃 ACTIVITY ⬭⬜⬜⬜⬭

📅 DATE		#️⃣ WEEK

💊 NAME	🌱 DOSAGE	🕐 TIME
		: AM / PM
		: AM / PM
		: AM / PM
		: AM / PM
		: AM / PM
		: AM / PM
		: AM / PM
		: AM / PM
		: AM / PM
		: AM / PM
		: AM / PM
		: AM / PM
		: AM / PM
		: AM / PM
		: AM / PM
		: AM / PM

🧠 SIDE EFFECTS	📝 ADDITIONAL NOTES
•	
•	
•	
•	
•	

PHYSICAL CONDITION

🌙 SLEEP	▭▭▭▭▭	🥤 WATER	▭▭▭▭▭
☀️ ENERGY	▭▭▭▭▭	🏃 ACTIVITY	▭▭▭▭▭

📅 DATE		# WEEK

💊 NAME	🌱 DOSAGE	🕐 TIME	
		:	AM / PM
		:	AM / PM
		:	AM / PM
		:	AM / PM
		:	AM / PM
		:	AM / PM
		:	AM / PM
		:	AM / PM
		:	AM / PM
		:	AM / PM
		:	AM / PM
		:	AM / PM
		:	AM / PM
		:	AM / PM
		:	AM / PM

🧠 SIDE EFFECTS	📝 ADDITIONAL NOTES
•	
•	
•	
•	
•	

PHYSICAL CONDITION	
🌙 SLEEP	🥛 WATER
⚡ ENERGY	🏃 ACTIVITY

📅 DATE	# WEEK

💊 NAME	🧪 DOSAGE	🕐 TIME
		: AM / PM
		: AM / PM
		: AM / PM
		: AM / PM
		: AM / PM
		: AM / PM
		: AM / PM
		: AM / PM
		: AM / PM
		: AM / PM
		: AM / PM
		: AM / PM
		: AM / PM
		: AM / PM
		: AM / PM

🤕 SIDE EFFECTS	📝 ADDITIONAL NOTES
•	
•	
•	
•	
•	

PHYSICAL CONDITION	
🌙 SLEEP ⬚⬚⬚⬚⬚	🥛 WATER ⬚⬚⬚⬚⬚
☀️ ENERGY ⬚⬚⬚⬚⬚	🏃 ACTIVITY ⬚⬚⬚⬚⬚

📅 DATE	# WEEK

💊 NAME	💊 DOSAGE	🕐 TIME	
		:	AM / PM
		:	AM / PM
		:	AM / PM
		:	AM / PM
		:	AM / PM
		:	AM / PM
		:	AM / PM
		:	AM / PM
		:	AM / PM
		:	AM / PM
		:	AM / PM
		:	AM / PM
		:	AM / PM
		:	AM / PM
		:	AM / PM

🤕 SIDE EFFECTS	📝 ADDITIONAL NOTES
•	
•	
•	
•	
•	

PHYSICAL CONDITION			
🌙 SLEEP	[ ][ ][ ][ ][ ]	🥤 WATER	[ ][ ][ ][ ][ ]
⚡ ENERGY	[ ][ ][ ][ ][ ]	🏃 ACTIVITY	[ ][ ][ ][ ][ ]

📅 DATE		#️⃣ WEEK

💊 NAME	💊 DOSAGE	🕐 TIME
		: AM / PM
		: AM / PM
		: AM / PM
		: AM / PM
		: AM / PM
		: AM / PM
		: AM / PM
		: AM / PM
		: AM / PM
		: AM / PM
		: AM / PM
		: AM / PM
		: AM / PM
		: AM / PM
		: AM / PM

🧠 SIDE EFFECTS	📝 ADDITIONAL NOTES
•	
•	
•	
•	
•	

PHYSICAL CONDITION	
🌙 SLEEP	🥤 WATER
⚡ ENERGY	🏃 ACTIVITY

📅 DATE		# WEEK

💊 NAME	💊 DOSAGE	⏱️ TIME	
		:	AM / PM
		:	AM / PM
		:	AM / PM
		:	AM / PM
		:	AM / PM
		:	AM / PM
		:	AM / PM
		:	AM / PM
		:	AM / PM
		:	AM / PM
		:	AM / PM
		:	AM / PM
		:	AM / PM
		:	AM / PM
		:	AM / PM

😷 SIDE EFFECTS	📝 ADDITIONAL NOTES
•	
•	
•	
•	
•	

PHYSICAL CONDITION	
🌙 SLEEP	🥛 WATER
🔆 ENERGY	🏃 ACTIVITY

📅 DATE		# WEEK

💊 NAME	🌱 DOSAGE	🕐 TIME
		: AM / PM
		: AM / PM
		: AM / PM
		: AM / PM
		: AM / PM
		: AM / PM
		: AM / PM
		: AM / PM
		: AM / PM
		: AM / PM
		: AM / PM
		: AM / PM
		: AM / PM
		: AM / PM
		: AM / PM

🧠 SIDE EFFECTS	📝 ADDITIONAL NOTES
•	
•	
•	
•	
•	

PHYSICAL CONDITION	
🌙 SLEEP ▭▭▭▭▭	🥛 WATER ▭▭▭▭▭
⚡ ENERGY ▭▭▭▭▭	🏃 ACTIVITY ▭▭▭▭▭

📅 DATE		# WEEK

💊 NAME	💊 DOSAGE	⏰ TIME
		: AM / PM
		: AM / PM
		: AM / PM
		: AM / PM
		: AM / PM
		: AM / PM
		: AM / PM
		: AM / PM
		: AM / PM
		: AM / PM
		: AM / PM
		: AM / PM
		: AM / PM
		: AM / PM
		: AM / PM

🗣 SIDE EFFECTS	📝 ADDITIONAL NOTES
•	
•	
•	
•	
•	

PHYSICAL CONDITION	
🌙 SLEEP ⬜⬜⬜⬜⬜	🥛 WATER ⬜⬜⬜⬜⬜
☀ ENERGY ⬜⬜⬜⬜⬜	🏃 ACTIVITY ⬜⬜⬜⬜⬜

DATE	# WEEK

🔖 NAME	💊 DOSAGE	⏰ TIME
		: AM / PM
		: AM / PM
		: AM / PM
		: AM / PM
		: AM / PM
		: AM / PM
		: AM / PM
		: AM / PM
		: AM / PM
		: AM / PM
		: AM / PM
		: AM / PM
		: AM / PM
		: AM / PM
		: AM / PM

🗣 SIDE EFFECTS	📝 ADDITIONAL NOTES
•	
•	
•	
•	
•	

PHYSICAL CONDITION	
🌙 SLEEP ⬡⬡⬡⬡⬡	🥛 WATER ⬡⬡⬡⬡⬡
⚡ ENERGY ⬡⬡⬡⬡⬡	🏃 ACTIVITY ⬡⬡⬡⬡⬡

📅 DATE		# WEEK

💊 NAME	🧪 DOSAGE	⏰ TIME
		: AM / PM
		: AM / PM
		: AM / PM
		: AM / PM
		: AM / PM
		: AM / PM
		: AM / PM
		: AM / PM
		: AM / PM
		: AM / PM
		: AM / PM
		: AM / PM
		: AM / PM
		: AM / PM
		: AM / PM

🧠 SIDE EFFECTS	📝 ADDITIONAL NOTES
•	
•	
•	
•	
•	

PHYSICAL CONDITION		
🌙 SLEEP	⬜⬜⬜⬜⬜	🥛 WATER ⬜⬜⬜⬜⬜
☀️ ENERGY	⬜⬜⬜⬜⬜	🏃 ACTIVITY ⬜⬜⬜⬜⬜

📅 DATE		#️⃣ WEEK

💊 NAME	🌱 DOSAGE	🕐 TIME
		: AM / PM
		: AM / PM
		: AM / PM
		: AM / PM
		: AM / PM
		: AM / PM
		: AM / PM
		: AM / PM
		: AM / PM
		: AM / PM
		: AM / PM
		: AM / PM
		: AM / PM
		: AM / PM
		: AM / PM
		: AM / PM

🧠 SIDE EFFECTS	📝 ADDITIONAL NOTES
•	
•	
•	
•	
•	

PHYSICAL CONDITION			
🌙 SLEEP	▭▭▭▭▭	🥛 WATER	▭▭▭▭▭
☀️ ENERGY	▭▭▭▭▭	🏃 ACTIVITY	▭▭▭▭▭

DATE		# WEEK

💊 NAME	🌱 DOSAGE	⏰ TIME
		: AM / PM
		: AM / PM
		: AM / PM
		: AM / PM
		: AM / PM
		: AM / PM
		: AM / PM
		: AM / PM
		: AM / PM
		: AM / PM
		: AM / PM
		: AM / PM
		: AM / PM
		: AM / PM
		: AM / PM

🤕 SIDE EFFECTS	📝 ADDITIONAL NOTES
•	
•	
•	
•	
•	

PHYSICAL CONDITION	
🌙 SLEEP	🥤 WATER
☀ ENERGY	🏃 ACTIVITY

📅 DATE		# WEEK

💊 NAME	💊 DOSAGE	🕐 TIME	
		:	AM / PM
		:	AM / PM
		:	AM / PM
		:	AM / PM
		:	AM / PM
		:	AM / PM
		:	AM / PM
		:	AM / PM
		:	AM / PM
		:	AM / PM
		:	AM / PM
		:	AM / PM
		:	AM / PM
		:	AM / PM
		:	AM / PM

🤕 SIDE EFFECTS	📝 ADDITIONAL NOTES
•	
•	
•	
•	
•	

PHYSICAL CONDITION	
🌙 SLEEP	🥛 WATER
⚡ ENERGY	🏃 ACTIVITY

📅 DATE		# WEEK

💊 NAME	💊 DOSAGE	🕐 TIME
		: AM / PM
		: AM / PM
		: AM / PM
		: AM / PM
		: AM / PM
		: AM / PM
		: AM / PM
		: AM / PM
		: AM / PM
		: AM / PM
		: AM / PM
		: AM / PM
		: AM / PM
		: AM / PM
		: AM / PM

🧠 SIDE EFFECTS	📝 ADDITIONAL NOTES
•	
•	
•	
•	
•	

PHYSICAL CONDITION	
🌙 SLEEP	🥛 WATER
⚡ ENERGY	🏃 ACTIVITY

📅 DATE		#️⃣ WEEK

💊 NAME	💊 DOSAGE	🕐 TIME
		: AM / PM
		: AM / PM
		: AM / PM
		: AM / PM
		: AM / PM
		: AM / PM
		: AM / PM
		: AM / PM
		: AM / PM
		: AM / PM
		: AM / PM
		: AM / PM
		: AM / PM
		: AM / PM
		: AM / PM

🤕 SIDE EFFECTS	📝 ADDITIONAL NOTES
•	
•	
•	
•	
•	

PHYSICAL CONDITION	
🌙 SLEEP	🥛 WATER
☀️ ENERGY	🏃 ACTIVITY

📅 DATE		# WEEK

💊 NAME	💊 DOSAGE	💊 TIME
		: AM / PM
		: AM / PM
		: AM / PM
		: AM / PM
		: AM / PM
		: AM / PM
		: AM / PM
		: AM / PM
		: AM / PM
		: AM / PM
		: AM / PM
		: AM / PM
		: AM / PM
		: AM / PM
		: AM / PM

🧑 SIDE EFFECTS	📝 ADDITIONAL NOTES
•	
•	
•	
•	
•	

PHYSICAL CONDITION	
🌙 SLEEP	🥤 WATER
⚡ ENERGY	🏃 ACTIVITY

📅 DATE		# WEEK

💊 NAME	💊 DOSAGE	🕐 TIME
		: AM / PM
		: AM / PM
		: AM / PM
		: AM / PM
		: AM / PM
		: AM / PM
		: AM / PM
		: AM / PM
		: AM / PM
		: AM / PM
		: AM / PM
		: AM / PM
		: AM / PM
		: AM / PM
		: AM / PM

🧠 SIDE EFFECTS	📝 ADDITIONAL NOTES
•	
•	
•	
•	
•	

PHYSICAL CONDITION	
🌙 SLEEP	🥛 WATER
⚡ ENERGY	🏃 ACTIVITY

📅 DATE		# WEEK	

💊 NAME	🌿 DOSAGE	⏱ TIME	
		:	AM / PM
		:	AM / PM
		:	AM / PM
		:	AM / PM
		:	AM / PM
		:	AM / PM
		:	AM / PM
		:	AM / PM
		:	AM / PM
		:	AM / PM
		:	AM / PM
		:	AM / PM
		:	AM / PM
		:	AM / PM
		:	AM / PM

🤕 SIDE EFFECTS	📝 ADDITIONAL NOTES
•	
•	
•	
•	
•	

PHYSICAL CONDITION			
🌙 SLEEP	⬜⬜⬜⬜	🥛 WATER	⬜⬜⬜⬜
⚡ ENERGY	⬜⬜⬜⬜	🏃 ACTIVITY	⬜⬜⬜⬜

📅 DATE		# WEEK

💊 NAME	🌱 DOSAGE	🕐 TIME
		: AM / PM
		: AM / PM
		: AM / PM
		: AM / PM
		: AM / PM
		: AM / PM
		: AM / PM
		: AM / PM
		: AM / PM
		: AM / PM
		: AM / PM
		: AM / PM
		: AM / PM
		: AM / PM
		: AM / PM

😷 SIDE EFFECTS	📝 ADDITIONAL NOTES
•	
•	
•	
•	
•	

PHYSICAL CONDITION	
🌙 SLEEP	🥛 WATER
⚡ ENERGY	🏃 ACTIVITY

📅 DATE		# WEEK

💊 NAME	💊 DOSAGE	🕐 TIME
		: AM / PM
		: AM / PM
		: AM / PM
		: AM / PM
		: AM / PM
		: AM / PM
		: AM / PM
		: AM / PM
		: AM / PM
		: AM / PM
		: AM / PM
		: AM / PM
		: AM / PM
		: AM / PM
		: AM / PM

🧑 SIDE EFFECTS	📝 ADDITIONAL NOTES
•	
•	
•	
•	
•	

PHYSICAL CONDITION	
🌙 SLEEP ☐☐☐☐☐	🥛 WATER ☐☐☐☐☐
☀ ENERGY ☐☐☐☐☐	🏃 ACTIVITY ☐☐☐☐☐

📅 DATE		# WEEK	

💊 NAME	🧴 DOSAGE	🕐 TIME	
		:	AM / PM
		:	AM / PM
		:	AM / PM
		:	AM / PM
		:	AM / PM
		:	AM / PM
		:	AM / PM
		:	AM / PM
		:	AM / PM
		:	AM / PM
		:	AM / PM
		:	AM / PM
		:	AM / PM
		:	AM / PM
		:	AM / PM

🧠 SIDE EFFECTS	📝 ADDITIONAL NOTES
•	
•	
•	
•	
•	

PHYSICAL CONDITION	
🌙 SLEEP	🥛 WATER
⚡ ENERGY	🏃 ACTIVITY

📅 DATE		# WEEK

💊 NAME	💊 DOSAGE	🕐 TIME
		: AM / PM
		: AM / PM
		: AM / PM
		: AM / PM
		: AM / PM
		: AM / PM
		: AM / PM
		: AM / PM
		: AM / PM
		: AM / PM
		: AM / PM
		: AM / PM
		: AM / PM
		: AM / PM
		: AM / PM

🧠 SIDE EFFECTS	📝 ADDITIONAL NOTES
•	
•	
•	
•	
•	

PHYSICAL CONDITION	
🌙 SLEEP ⬜⬜⬜⬜⬜	🥛 WATER ⬜⬜⬜⬜⬜
⚡ ENERGY ⬜⬜⬜⬜⬜	🏃 ACTIVITY ⬜⬜⬜⬜⬜

📅 DATE		# WEEK

💊 NAME	🌱 DOSAGE	🕐 TIME
		: AM / PM
		: AM / PM
		: AM / PM
		: AM / PM
		: AM / PM
		: AM / PM
		: AM / PM
		: AM / PM
		: AM / PM
		: AM / PM
		: AM / PM
		: AM / PM
		: AM / PM
		: AM / PM
		: AM / PM

🧠 SIDE EFFECTS	📝 ADDITIONAL NOTES
•	
•	
•	
•	
•	

PHYSICAL CONDITION			
🌙 SLEEP	⬜⬜⬜⬜⬜	🥤 WATER	⬜⬜⬜⬜⬜
⚡ ENERGY	⬜⬜⬜⬜⬜	🏃 ACTIVITY	⬜⬜⬜⬜⬜

📅 DATE		# WEEK

💊 NAME	🌡 DOSAGE	⏰ TIME
		: AM / PM
		: AM / PM
		: AM / PM
		: AM / PM
		: AM / PM
		: AM / PM
		: AM / PM
		: AM / PM
		: AM / PM
		: AM / PM
		: AM / PM
		: AM / PM
		: AM / PM
		: AM / PM
		: AM / PM

🧠 SIDE EFFECTS	📝 ADDITIONAL NOTES
•	
•	
•	
•	
•	

PHYSICAL CONDITION	
🌙 SLEEP ▭▭▭▭▭	🥛 WATER ▭▭▭▭▭
☀ ENERGY ▭▭▭▭▭	🏃 ACTIVITY ▭▭▭▭▭

📅 DATE		# WEEK

💊 NAME	🌱 DOSAGE	🕐 TIME
		: AM / PM
		: AM / PM
		: AM / PM
		: AM / PM
		: AM / PM
		: AM / PM
		: AM / PM
		: AM / PM
		: AM / PM
		: AM / PM
		: AM / PM
		: AM / PM
		: AM / PM
		: AM / PM
		: AM / PM

🧑 SIDE EFFECTS	📝 ADDITIONAL NOTES
•	
•	
•	
•	
•	

PHYSICAL CONDITION	
🌙 SLEEP	💧 WATER
⚡ ENERGY	🏃 ACTIVITY

📅 DATE		# WEEK	

💊 NAME	🌱 DOSAGE	🕐 TIME	
		:	AM / PM
		:	AM / PM
		:	AM / PM
		:	AM / PM
		:	AM / PM
		:	AM / PM
		:	AM / PM
		:	AM / PM
		:	AM / PM
		:	AM / PM
		:	AM / PM
		:	AM / PM
		:	AM / PM
		:	AM / PM

🧠 SIDE EFFECTS	📝 ADDITIONAL NOTES
•	
•	
•	
•	
•	

PHYSICAL CONDITION			
☾ SLEEP	⬚⬚⬚⬚⬚	🥛 WATER	⬚⬚⬚⬚⬚
☀ ENERGY	⬚⬚⬚⬚⬚	🏃 ACTIVITY	⬚⬚⬚⬚⬚

📅 DATE	# WEEK

💊 NAME	💊 DOSAGE	🕐 TIME
		: AM / PM
		: AM / PM
		: AM / PM
		: AM / PM
		: AM / PM
		: AM / PM
		: AM / PM
		: AM / PM
		: AM / PM
		: AM / PM
		: AM / PM
		: AM / PM
		: AM / PM
		: AM / PM
		: AM / PM

🤕 SIDE EFFECTS	📝 ADDITIONAL NOTES
•	
•	
•	
•	
•	

PHYSICAL CONDITION			
🌙 SLEEP	⬡⬡⬡⬡⬡	🥛 WATER	⬡⬡⬡⬡⬡
⚡ ENERGY	⬡⬡⬡⬡⬡	🏃 ACTIVITY	⬡⬡⬡⬡⬡

📅 DATE		# WEEK

💊 NAME	🥣 DOSAGE	🕐 TIME
		: AM / PM
		: AM / PM
		: AM / PM
		: AM / PM
		: AM / PM
		: AM / PM
		: AM / PM
		: AM / PM
		: AM / PM
		: AM / PM
		: AM / PM
		: AM / PM
		: AM / PM
		: AM / PM
		: AM / PM
		: AM / PM

🧠 SIDE EFFECTS	📝 ADDITIONAL NOTES
•	
•	
•	
•	
•	

PHYSICAL CONDITION	
🌙 SLEEP ⬭▭▭▭⬭	🥛 WATER ⬭▭▭▭⬭
⚡ ENERGY ⬭▭▭▭⬭	🏃 ACTIVITY ⬭▭▭▭⬭

📅 DATE	#️⃣ WEEK

💊 NAME	💊 DOSAGE	🕐 TIME	
		:	AM / PM
		:	AM / PM
		:	AM / PM
		:	AM / PM
		:	AM / PM
		:	AM / PM
		:	AM / PM
		:	AM / PM
		:	AM / PM
		:	AM / PM
		:	AM / PM
		:	AM / PM
		:	AM / PM
		:	AM / PM
		:	AM / PM

🗯 SIDE EFFECTS	📝 ADDITIONAL NOTES
•	
•	
•	
•	
•	

PHYSICAL CONDITION	
🌙 SLEEP	🥛 WATER
☀ ENERGY	🏃 ACTIVITY

📅 DATE		# WEEK

💊 NAME	🧴 DOSAGE	⏰ TIME	
		:	AM / PM
		:	AM / PM
		:	AM / PM
		:	AM / PM
		:	AM / PM
		:	AM / PM
		:	AM / PM
		:	AM / PM
		:	AM / PM
		:	AM / PM
		:	AM / PM
		:	AM / PM
		:	AM / PM
		:	AM / PM
		:	AM / PM

🤕 SIDE EFFECTS	📝 ADDITIONAL NOTES
•	
•	
•	
•	
•	

PHYSICAL CONDITION			
🌙 SLEEP	⬭⬭⬭⬭⬭	🥤 WATER	⬭⬭⬭⬭⬭
⚡ ENERGY	⬭⬭⬭⬭⬭	🏃 ACTIVITY	⬭⬭⬭⬭⬭

📅 DATE		#️⃣ WEEK

💊 NAME	🪴 DOSAGE	🕐 TIME
		: AM / PM
		: AM / PM
		: AM / PM
		: AM / PM
		: AM / PM
		: AM / PM
		: AM / PM
		: AM / PM
		: AM / PM
		: AM / PM
		: AM / PM
		: AM / PM
		: AM / PM
		: AM / PM
		: AM / PM

🤕 SIDE EFFECTS	📝 ADDITIONAL NOTES
•	
•	
•	
•	
•	

PHYSICAL CONDITION		
🌙 SLEEP	▭▭▭▭▭	🥛 WATER ▭▭▭▭▭
⚡ ENERGY	▭▭▭▭▭	🏃 ACTIVITY ▭▭▭▭▭

📅 DATE		# WEEK

💊 NAME	💊 DOSAGE	🕐 TIME
		: AM / PM
		: AM / PM
		: AM / PM
		: AM / PM
		: AM / PM
		: AM / PM
		: AM / PM
		: AM / PM
		: AM / PM
		: AM / PM
		: AM / PM
		: AM / PM
		: AM / PM
		: AM / PM
		: AM / PM

🤕 SIDE EFFECTS	📝 ADDITIONAL NOTES
•	
•	
•	
•	
•	

PHYSICAL CONDITION	
🌙 SLEEP ⬜⬜⬜⬜⬜	🥛 WATER ⬜⬜⬜⬜⬜
☀️ ENERGY ⬜⬜⬜⬜⬜	🏃 ACTIVITY ⬜⬜⬜⬜⬜

📅 DATE		# WEEK

💊 NAME	💊 DOSAGE	🕐 TIME
		: AM / PM
		: AM / PM
		: AM / PM
		: AM / PM
		: AM / PM
		: AM / PM
		: AM / PM
		: AM / PM
		: AM / PM
		: AM / PM
		: AM / PM
		: AM / PM
		: AM / PM
		: AM / PM
		: AM / PM

🧠 SIDE EFFECTS	📝 ADDITIONAL NOTES
•	
•	
•	
•	
•	

PHYSICAL CONDITION	
🌙 SLEEP	🥛 WATER
⚡ ENERGY	🏃 ACTIVITY

📅 DATE	# WEEK

💊 NAME	🪴 DOSAGE	⏰ TIME	
		:	AM / PM
		:	AM / PM
		:	AM / PM
		:	AM / PM
		:	AM / PM
		:	AM / PM
		:	AM / PM
		:	AM / PM
		:	AM / PM
		:	AM / PM
		:	AM / PM
		:	AM / PM
		:	AM / PM
		:	AM / PM
		:	AM / PM

🧠 SIDE EFFECTS	📝 ADDITIONAL NOTES
•	
•	
•	
•	
•	

PHYSICAL CONDITION

🌙 SLEEP		🥤 WATER	
⚡ ENERGY		🏃 ACTIVITY	

📅 DATE		# WEEK

💊 NAME	🌿 DOSAGE	🕐 TIME
		: AM / PM
		: AM / PM
		: AM / PM
		: AM / PM
		: AM / PM
		: AM / PM
		: AM / PM
		: AM / PM
		: AM / PM
		: AM / PM
		: AM / PM
		: AM / PM
		: AM / PM
		: AM / PM
		: AM / PM
		: AM / PM

🗣 SIDE EFFECTS	📝 ADDITIONAL NOTES
•	
•	
•	
•	
•	

PHYSICAL CONDITION			
🌙 SLEEP	▭▭▭▭▭	🥤 WATER	▭▭▭▭▭
⚡ ENERGY	▭▭▭▭▭	🏃 ACTIVITY	▭▭▭▭▭

📅 DATE		# WEEK

💊 NAME	🧴 DOSAGE	⏰ TIME
		: AM / PM
		: AM / PM
		: AM / PM
		: AM / PM
		: AM / PM
		: AM / PM
		: AM / PM
		: AM / PM
		: AM / PM
		: AM / PM
		: AM / PM
		: AM / PM
		: AM / PM
		: AM / PM
		: AM / PM

🤕 SIDE EFFECTS	📝 ADDITIONAL NOTES
•	
•	
•	
•	
•	

PHYSICAL CONDITION	
🌙 SLEEP ⬭⬭⬭⬭⬭	🥛 WATER ⬭⬭⬭⬭⬭
⚡ ENERGY ⬭⬭⬭⬭⬭	🏃 ACTIVITY ⬭⬭⬭⬭⬭

📅 DATE	# WEEK

💊 NAME	🌡 DOSAGE	⏰ TIME
		: AM / PM
		: AM / PM
		: AM / PM
		: AM / PM
		: AM / PM
		: AM / PM
		: AM / PM
		: AM / PM
		: AM / PM
		: AM / PM
		: AM / PM
		: AM / PM
		: AM / PM
		: AM / PM
		: AM / PM

🧑 SIDE EFFECTS	📝 ADDITIONAL NOTES
•	
•	
•	
•	
•	

PHYSICAL CONDITION		
🌙 SLEEP	▭▭▭▭▭	🥛 WATER ▭▭▭▭▭
☀ ENERGY	▭▭▭▭▭	🏃 ACTIVITY ▭▭▭▭▭

📅 DATE		# WEEK	

💊 NAME	🌱 DOSAGE	🕐 TIME	
		:	AM / PM
		:	AM / PM
		:	AM / PM
		:	AM / PM
		:	AM / PM
		:	AM / PM
		:	AM / PM
		:	AM / PM
		:	AM / PM
		:	AM / PM
		:	AM / PM
		:	AM / PM
		:	AM / PM
		:	AM / PM
		:	AM / PM

🧠 SIDE EFFECTS	📝 ADDITIONAL NOTES
•	
•	
•	
•	
•	

PHYSICAL CONDITION			
🌙 SLEEP	⬜⬜⬜⬜⬜	🥛 WATER	⬜⬜⬜⬜⬜
⚡ ENERGY	⬜⬜⬜⬜⬜	🏃 ACTIVITY	⬜⬜⬜⬜⬜

📅 DATE		# WEEK

💊 NAME	🌱 DOSAGE	🕐 TIME
		: AM / PM
		: AM / PM
		: AM / PM
		: AM / PM
		: AM / PM
		: AM / PM
		: AM / PM
		: AM / PM
		: AM / PM
		: AM / PM
		: AM / PM
		: AM / PM
		: AM / PM
		: AM / PM
		: AM / PM

🤕 SIDE EFFECTS	📝 ADDITIONAL NOTES
•	
•	
•	
•	
•	

PHYSICAL CONDITION	
🌙 SLEEP	🥛 WATER
⚡ ENERGY	🏃 ACTIVITY

📅 DATE		# WEEK

💊 NAME	🧴 DOSAGE	🕐 TIME
		: AM / PM
		: AM / PM
		: AM / PM
		: AM / PM
		: AM / PM
		: AM / PM
		: AM / PM
		: AM / PM
		: AM / PM
		: AM / PM
		: AM / PM
		: AM / PM
		: AM / PM
		: AM / PM
		: AM / PM

🧠 SIDE EFFECTS	📝 ADDITIONAL NOTES
•	
•	
•	
•	
•	

PHYSICAL CONDITION	
🌙 SLEEP ⬜⬜⬜⬜⬜	🥛 WATER ⬜⬜⬜⬜⬜
⚡ ENERGY ⬜⬜⬜⬜⬜	🏃 ACTIVITY ⬜⬜⬜⬜⬜

📅 DATE	# WEEK

💊 NAME	🌿 DOSAGE	🕐 TIME
		: AM / PM
		: AM / PM
		: AM / PM
		: AM / PM
		: AM / PM
		: AM / PM
		: AM / PM
		: AM / PM
		: AM / PM
		: AM / PM
		: AM / PM
		: AM / PM
		: AM / PM
		: AM / PM
		: AM / PM

🧑 SIDE EFFECTS	📝 ADDITIONAL NOTES
•	
•	
•	
•	
•	

PHYSICAL CONDITION	
🌙 SLEEP	🥛 WATER
⚡ ENERGY	🏃 ACTIVITY

www.ingramcontent.com/pod-product-compliance
Lightning Source LLC
Chambersburg PA
CBHW051033030426
42336CB00015B/2849